1

Printed in the United States of America.

Flowers Book Series

Email: flowersbookseries@gmail.com

Library of Congress Cataloging-in-Publication Data.

ISBN-13: 978-1500540913

ISBN-10: 1500540919

I'm a Caregiver!

Who said this was easy.

By

Mary K. Hukill

.....a humorous look at my Journey.

Dedicated to My Mom

Dorothy F. Wolford

In Honor and Memory to

Dr. Romelle A. Belmonte

We wouldn't be here at this moment without your help. Amen.

THANKS! To

My Brother, *Ellis Perry Hukill, III*

Introduction

Tsk, Tsk......I Won the Lottery! I get to
Caregive for my Mom. You may say,
"what? Isn't that a lot of work?".
YES!!! It most certainly is. But, my
Mom is still alive. A lot of others don't
have their Mom alive, let alone their
Father, Step-Mother, or Step-Father.
So, I Won the Lottery! I get to spend
time with my Mom, sure, we disagree,
have simple arguments, like different
yet the same in foods, certainly read
different types of books, and have
other taste, style, and interest
differences. What we have in common
is the understanding is that you help
your other Family members the Best
way you can and know how to do. Be

there to help one another. Who else is going to do it.

As a Caregiver, whether for yourself, your Parent, Family Relative, or, a Friend be a Health Advocate. You do matter. Keep track of what is going on and make sure what needs to happen, does.

Are you READY!!!

Caregiving isn't for Sissies………..What are you doing here!

If you think that Cotton Candy, Carmel Apples, and Hot Apple Cider is furnished at this Rodeo ride, think again. You will be Lucky! That your teeth are still in your head and you have your wits about you when doing the Caregiving gig. This isn't a Pony ride. It can be at moments, when you 'think' you have it all together and you find out that you did indeed miss something, forgot something, didn't turn the lights off, forgot your keys, where are the Insurance cards, who turned off the stove or oven, and, who will pick up the UPS package left at the Front Door during a huge downpour. Folks, and, this is just in an hour or two of work Caregiving. I found out that I have to plan ahead, write a LOT of notes where I need to be, when I need to be there, WHAT is it that I bring to any appointments. You now are the Caregiving Concierge. Your thoughts are how to keep things in order for another person. Buckle Up! Buttercups. Until you grasp the true situation...you will flounder, be frustrated, and NOT have any way to work this to your advantage.

Being a Caregiver doesn't mean you are a Prisoner.

Be sure to realize, you are not dead, yet. You must somehow enjoy! The outside World. Get away some times, learn to have others or paid help watch over who you are Caregiving so that you can occasionally do something different. If you don't, in my Opinion, you have given over your Life to someone else, you are NOT living your Life, you are in the 'walking dead zone'. Get out of that. Sure, you want to help Caregive. But, if you don't take care of yourself, you will soon be in no position to be too helpful to some one else.

I always tell my Mom that there needs to be time for me to see what is going on in the Marketplace so that I can see the changes and react to them. Plus, I need to find out what Stores have changed what so that I can purchase items at the best value and know where they can be purchased. Don't assume all stores sell all sizes and products. Draw up a plan, work the plan, now seize the Day! And make good things happen. Sometimes you get Lucky along the way! There could be Sales in stores not mentioned, sometimes we find prices are lower than expected, there are new Stores popping up, some Stores close, and, there are other myriad reasons to always keep yourself aware of what is

going on in the world. Your world.
Things change.   Constantly.

Also, be a human being. If you want to
see a Concert Event, a Movie, or a
special show, you need to get out of
the four walls and explore. Be a
Human. Find someone to fill in for a
bit, hey, the person you are caregiving
needs change also. Sure, you can find
a FREE Video or CD Movie at the local
Library and bring it back and watch it.
When possible, let yourself have some
FREE time to see things, experience
some FRESH things in Life. Life must
be lived. It isn't for the Dead, and, you
are not dead, yet. Live Life. You may
once a week take a class of some
subject just to unwind. You must

refresh your batteries. You won't be any good to anyone else, let alone yourself if you don't STOP for a moment, and live Life. End of Sermon.

Your Food and their Food.

There will be times when a Doctor will stipulate to the one you are caring for some practical foods to either eat or to NOT eat. The Foods that are NOT good for them may be due to swallowing, calories, certain attributes the food has, or, what it can do to someone, and various other reasons. Listen to the Doctor. It may not always make sense to you, but, read up on it, or think it out and you will soon possibly agree to the suggestions made. Do be aware that you don't have to always agree with any Doctor. They didn't come down from the Mountain Top with some Tablets with medical rules written, enscribed, or delegated to be the Final "word" on things. Use your mind, have some sense about you and be wise. What works works. What doesn't work won't.

It is all right to make mistakes as long as it doesn't affect the safety, well being, or, life of the one you are helping. They don't think right when on Medication, sometimes age is a factor, and, knowledge. Do the best you can, research on the internet, ask the Pharmacist, call the Doctor's office when you need. If there is a "My Chart" or some website program the Doctors office or Hospital uses---that can be a great tool to help you and the Doctor understand medical conditions. Use the practical help. It saves time, gets to a discussion to find an answer, and, allows a more thorough way to follow health issues and updates.

The Airport and all those Cards for body replacements.

My Family teases my Mom that she is the new Bionic Woman. Parts is parts in her Life. And, if she could, I'd say she'd replace a few more to function even better. As you get older, you may not be able to replace more parts. Knee replacements and Pacemakers are new items you want others to know that are there.

Do remember to ask the Doctor after a "parts" surgery to have the Cards stating you have certain materials now in their Body. You don't want to go through Federal Building or Airport Check Points sounding off the Alarms, literally. It may be "FUN!" or Exciting for the moment, but, with your Doctor office giving you these new cards of information, it also helps any Emergency Medical staff know ahead of time what they may be dealing with. If someone has other Medical conditions that needs a bracelet, necklace, or just hanging on some chain, it is advisable to have any pertinent Medical information around. Mom has lists in her special coin and dollar purse, that fits inside any purse she has, various Medical cards, Insurance cards, Library card, and what other information she needs. Neighbor phone numbers, Family phone numbers, her Attorney is written out on note pages, or, can be 3 X 5 notecards folded what is needed if ever needed. It is organized, tight having some rubber band around some items, and is easy to reach at the Doctor office. People appreciate it when there is that kind of order and organization. Be a Solution and not the problem. Help the Health folks that want to help you.

Lollipops and Candy.

My Mom has an infinity for Chocolate and good Lollipops. She will clobber you silly and reach across a table if any piece of Chocolate is nearing hitting the floor. It is like a wild crazy dance leaping over the Table top to make sure that even one small lump of Candy doesn't touch the Floor. The dainty Ballet lunge is Quite fascinating. She has trouble with her legs or knees every so often to do errands, but, doesn't miss a beat to save any Chocolate. It is a horrible day when any Chocolate has to hit the trash can. Bummer.

Now, when Baking, she uses only Butter, and, you have to have the BEST possible Chocolate Chips. Otherwise, it isn't being baked. Mom has her likes and dislikes, but, anything Chocolate, even Chocolate Tea, is her domain. We both love Chocolate Coffee. Who doesn't. Chocolate can sooth the tired soul, calm nerves, and amend offenses.

Lollipops are great to fetch while at the local Bank and bring to the car and give to the 'child' , your Mom, and she purrs like a satisfied cat, Life is Good when there are Lollipops and Chocolate.

Folks may lose their taste as they get older.

I'm not sure why this attribute happens, but, as people age, they sometimes lose their taste. Food isn't as attractive to them. No Zip. No Tangy. No Special Sauce to wake up those taste buds. Adjust. Don't complain, whine, or, find reasons not to eat. What folks can taste is what they can taste. If there are situations to be aware of, then, contact your Doctor and explain any changes. Food is GOOD to eat when well prepared, the right dish, and something the person you are helping likes to eat. And, sometimes, their tastes for certain foods may change, every so often, and, back again. Just Adjust. Go forward.

Find some Food items you both can enjoy. Sometimes, I make two different Turkey Dressings to fit all folks dietary needs or food tastes. That is a minor thing to do and is greatly appreciated. With the various Grocery products that are constantly being updated and upgrades, there is always plenty of options for you and who you give care. Find some Balance.

Splurge once in a while, when you can.

Purchase that extra flower package to plant. Purchase some neat eats from the bakery or have some tasty pizza once in a while.

No one has a timeline when each of us can pass away. So Enjoy! something neat once in a while. You should find small ways to brighten up your day since you are the one coordinating everything to function well. While all of this Caregiving is happening, Life is going by. You need to experience things as they come, when they come, and as they come. If you just do the wash, clean the floors, wipe out the trashcan, then, that is all Life will be about to you during this phase. You must find the small things to enjoy along the way.

Savor some brand new line of Coffee, have some Marshmallows in your Hot Chocolate, add some new flavoring to your hot Tea, add some Mint or Peppermint to your Iced Tea, try a new recipe that all can enjoy, if a new restaurant opens have a side dish or entrée to serve, and do smell the Roses when along the way where they are growing. Make the Day more like Living!

Going for walks at 9:30pm and at 1:00am and 2:00am.

My Mom had Back Surgery and that Summer it was a HOT Temperature time in the Midwest. Eggs sure could have been fried in a skillet in any Parking Lot. It was HOT! The steam was so thick it was difficult to breathe even for a normal healthy person, let alone someone that just had Back Surgery. There was no Question that Mom had to walk to bring up her strength. But, the heat was so bad and the neighbors were not going to understand that their Germs were not welcome.

So, my Mom and I did her walking excercises about 9:30pm, or, at

10:00pm, just about every night. Sometimes if we were both up we'd go around 1:00am or even at 3:00am. We walked when possible, around the sidewalk and parking lot, Mom used her walker and slowly got more energy, could breathe better, and we didn't have Germs from any one else trying to help.

The Walking Dead.

Some days it can seem like all you are being is the Walking Dead. You do the same things over and over, and over, again, and nothing good and positive about Life is helping you. You don't seem to have anything new to wake up and make you Excited about Life or even living. Well, dust off that attitude right now, and change things. You have to change things every so often, turn things on its side and redo, add in something GOOD for you to enjoy! And learn that tomorrow is another day. Life does go on.

You may need to add some new faces in your schedule to help Caregive. Call another relative or two and see when they can take over and bring in a meal, go out to eat and let you stay Home to do something YOU want to do or finish up doing. Call your Church to send some Volunteers to sit with a loved one. Call on a Non-Profit group that helps sit with folks so that you can Shop or go to your own Doctor Appointments. You are not Superman or Superwoman. You can wear a Cape, but, don't let it overcome what you can or can't do. Learn to delegate, make lists of what YOU also need to accomplish in a day, and find a way to make that Happen. No, it isn't easy. There may be frustration that you are not keeping court all the time in 'their' needs. So, what. Find a way to plow forward and recapture what is really about livng your Life in a now restricted way of Life. Make a balance of how you can change things around and include what you want to do every so often. If you haven't done that, or, feel that you can't then change things. If you don't you have lost the battles and certainly the war. You have lost your Life for someone else. What about YOUR Life. It matters. Now, find a way to show something each day, when possible, what you are all about, what your Destiny is, and how are you getting there. It is step by step, piece by piece. In time, you will see a major change and possible condition. It all adds up. Now, start building the pieces.

The Hospital Floor looks good waxed and clean—how about the rest of the Hospital.

When you have the chance to wait at the Hospital at a Surgery, before a Doctor comes in, between the Nurse duties, you may have a LOT of time sitting, waiting, fretting, praying, going between various Medical Departments. I look at the Floor quite a bit. It is there, I'm looking around and I see the Floor. You can learn a lot looking at the Floor where you are. And, sometimes is is good and sometimes it isn't.

I always thanked whoever was cleaning or waxing the Hospital floor as it may be the cleanest area in your Hospital.

Ask Questions when folks change your linens—ask for them to be changed if they need it. When and how do you clean the private Hospital room restroom. Who cleans the commode and how often. You need to take charge of the area around you. Bacteria can creep up like a song---and, you better be the band leader. Otherwise, infections can rule the day and sometimes can cause Death. All you need is one infection to cause problems. Don't assume a Hospital is the cleanest place on earth. It isn't, some of the time. Now, one Hospital that my Mom and I go to you can possibly, sit on their Floors and eat off of them. They are impressive clean no matter what hallway, room, area we are. We're Blessed on coming to this particular Health Facility. Now, not every situation is peachy clean at any facility. Cloth seats in chairs can carry Bacteria at your Doctor office. Look for a leather or vinyl chair to sit in. Clean off any Table Top with your package of Alcohol wipes you now keep in a purse or bag you bring with you everywhere. Don't care about hurting someone elses 'feelings'. Learn that only one infection can take you down, or you loved one. My Mom was Blessed with 5, yes, count them 5 Bacteria after a surgery. My Aunt, at the same timeframe contracted only One Bacteria, went through her pelvis bone into her body and she later passed away. My Aunt only went to a swank Hospital for a procedure, went Home, didn't feel good, got some bacteria, and within two weeks passed away from it. My Mom was Lucky from her attitude, her newfound friend a Bacteria Doctor, some experimental type drugs, and lots of Daily visits for infusions to the Hospital and then to the Doctor office. Daily. It was four to six hours a day to do this. I first asked if the Ambulance ride could take her, which could happen, but, one Doctor felt to cut down more contracting Bacteria, me or someone else was to take her. Well, we did. Three of us split up the week and drove where we needed. If the Hospital or the Doctor Office was ready for us we got the procedure over in a few hours. If not, we were there for many hours just to get hooked up for a Transfusion. Sure, Mom had two infusions at first.

I read on the internet for us to increase the amount of Vegetables, Fruits, add more nuts to the diet, protein, and the magic of it all, in my Opinion was to have yogurt at least once a day. Now, to me, that is the Magic sauce. We already ate well, did increase eating more varieties of nuts, and did add yogurt. To this day, both of us do not go through the day without having our dose of yogurt. Be creative in what brand you want. I have a neat plain vanilla pudding type and it is the magic sauce. It keeps your system running, cleans out whatever, and makes you feel as though, in time, you are doing the right thing for your body. It is the Magic sauce, in my Opinion. You have to do all the other foods, but, once a day, is the way, to this day! Amen.

We were Lucky! That mom came out of that ordeal. It was a year and a half later of rest, that former situation took us almost a year to get past also, and another year to work up her strength. It was about 3 years to get past that Surgery, the next surgery to cut out Bacteria on some body fat that fortunately didn't affect any other body tissue or organ, and, then resting up to have more body strength.   That alone, was an ordeal. And, we were Lucky her body came out of that. It was a horrible, time consuming ordeal, a tough road to tow, and I'm glad I made it out alive. We washed everything we could, as fast as possible, kept dusting, cleaning, and cleaning again, and washed what ever items needed to be kept clean. THAT was also key to survival.

Yes, be aware of your Hospital surroundings. It will help you live or not live. Don't assume that 'they' are the answer. They are the ones to watch to help keep the Hospital clean. Tell them on survey cards what you saw that needed to be cleaned. They are more than happy to help. Your Life and who you are Caregiving will depend on this. Clean, clean, clean. Is it clean.

Pets of some sort can help calm folks.

Some folks have pets. We're not into pets at this time of my Mom's life. I'm not good at making sure pets are cared for as much as helping Mom. I can do Gold Fish or a Whispering Willow Tree. Anything else, even some stuffed animals are not in my DNA to keep alive, too well. Mom kept the Family cats alive, fed, and took them to the Vet when it was their last days.

If you can take care of pets and want to do that also, it is your call. I'd not be a good indicator on this one. Family pets can help keep folks blood pressure low. They can be good to keep folks calm. They do the opposite for me. If you can bring in the pets to your Caregiving experience, Good Luck! Do what you feel will help them. If it means finding a service to bring in a pet type animal, to pet, feed, or brush their coats, then, I'm for it. What you feel will make the ones you Caregive feel better, make their lives a well rounded phase, and, help give you more good experiences then go for it. Do feed your pets.

Alcohol wipes are one of your new Best Friends.

Accept it.   The World can get pretty dirty out there. Who knows what you live in, but, the outside World can become a festival of Bacteria. You work hard to NOT contract an infection. Sometimes the odds are against you and you just have to roll with the punches. Learn that you can fight back and hopefully win. No matter if it is the Flu season, in the Summer, you need to have, in my Opinion, some Alcohol wipes in the Trunk of your car, in the car glove compartment, all over rooms or a central room where you are living or staying. Reach for an alcohol wipe to keep your hands clean, be clean. Sure, I wash my hands a lot when touching certain medical needs, any help with bodily fluids, and medicine. You need to be clean. I can not overstate this enough. Alcohol wipes can Quickly wipe off counter tops, commodes, hands, and other needs immediately. Be safe, be clean, and be wise. Clean is Best.

Bacteria is everywhere and you are stuck where you are.

Don't ever assume that you will be safe from having infections from Bacteria the Hospital or Doctor Office may have. Infections can happen for various reasons. Be aware to keep your hands clean, wash off anything you have a 'feeling' about, and watch how clean the restrooms are.

My Aunt passed away being at a Brand new Hospital, considered 'swank' from its location and new Technology. Things can happen. The right situation can have that creepy Bacteria creep into your body for various reasons that just allow it to happen and travel fast.

Bacteria is bad, can cause horrible problems, and even Death.

Good Luck! Sometimes, it is the Luck of the draw, what has happened with your Body, how strong you are and how healthy you are. Just realize that you have to Fight. Always Fight. Have the right Attitude. Attitude is important. Get the right one!

Didn't need that Surgery!

My Mom was so sick from one Surgery…..high temperature, not too responsive, etc. It was above what I could do and wanted to do. Sometimes you have to know your capable limits.

An ambulance was called and we both went to the local Hospital ER. I like the ER as the Doctors are very FAST on what trauma has happened. Mom and I were tired from her last Surgery, flat out. She had some X-Rays, had a horrible high temperature and was considered very sick. At that time, we didn't know she had so many Bacteria infections. Well, some Doctors had thought she needed another surgery in her abdomen but it was decided not to do anything. The ER Doctors thought the same thing. They wanted to do Surgery in a few hours. We were so tired.....we muttered....kinda' like.....sure, all righttttt, okayyyyyy, whateverrrrr.....tone. Well, in a half an hour later, they reread the X-Rays and also agreed the Surgery wasn't needed. And, here we were ready to do this. UGH. THANKS! to all the ER Doctors that looked at it, again, and saw that some other area was in the way to make the best decision. At least they were man enough to do that. We appreciated that. We were so tired. I'm Thankful that God does watch over us and help via others to do the right thing. Sure, it could have easily been that Mom was soon going to be prepped for another Surgery she didn't need, yet. I'm just glad that we didn't have to do something that wasn't needed, in actuality. Ever. I'm sure that she'd ask her Family Physician before doing anything, anyway, but, she was very sick and something had to be done. Who knows how that may have happened, but, it work out, Thankfully.

She did later, a few days more have to undergo a Surgery to get rid of some Bacteria and that went rather well. It was making her sick, otherwise. Now, that Surgery she needed, whether she liked it or not.

If the Neighbors need some help from their children, then, call for help!

My Mom's Neighbors are over the age of 55 where she lives. And, they need help sometimes. Some go to Assisted Living, some move in with their children, and some had needed to live closer to their kids and actually move out of State. It is what it is. As folks age they may need various changes in how others need to know what help they need. Be a Solution and not a Problem.

When we saw that a couple living next door were really way past needing some Family help, my Mom called, per my suggestion, and told their Children what we were seeing. Now, all situations are different. This particular situation soon prompted help from their kids we hadn't seen before. It was needed. If you see the day to day situations of folks and know they need more help, do find help. In this situation, it was two 80 years olds that were overcome with the Quality of Life they could do from how age strips folks of what they can do in helping another individual. All of a sudden, it was both folks working to survive aging. And, it wasn't fair that the Lady of the House had to work to help the Man of the House move from chair to chair lifting him. It was hard to know, and, when needing help, called for us to help her. She had lost a lot of weight and had to purchase a lot of new clothes. She looked great, but, to lose weight that way was horrible to see.

When you can help folks, great, and how much time you can do that. Some folks appreciate it and some folks don't. Do ONLY what you can. Don't do anything more. It isn't YOUR fight. But, do call someone about what you are aware. Now, realize that some Family members do NOT want to be bothered. You just have to realize that. Hopefully, you will reach the right person to help. If not, just do what you can. It isn't your Family member. There is stress and strain taking care of others and you don't need the extra amount on your shoulders. It will affect your body,

your mind, and possibly your Spirit.
Don't take on the World. You need to
survive. If you go down, then what.

It is always the little things that count in Life.

What counts is the little things to help brighten up folks lives. This can be a flower from the Garden. Place several chocolate pieces in a sack or baggie and give to someone. You can help with the Bags of Groceries from the car. Wash someone's car, drive someone to their Doctor appointment or to Church. Be there to listen to the same old story or news, again, again about an event that seems important to that person. Wipe off crumbs on another persons face or shirt. Open the door for someone. Be there when they need you at a serious moment and need a shoulder to cry on. Be the person who stood up for another during a trying time or unfair moment. Know when to stop by a Business owned by a friend who needs help from a staff member not showing up that day.

What you do in the smallest of moments count the most. Sure, it is Great! To win an Award or new Client. It is more important that you were there to lift someone up who needed it that Day!

Bring Flowers in for the Table...good for the Soul.

When it is Spring I get very excited to find out what new Flowers have made it to the various store shelves. In doing errands, it is not out of the ordinary for me to also drive past some store areas where the mulch, rock, and soon to be more Flowers sit. I wait with Great expectantcy. My Mom loves Flowers. I wait to see what new beautiful flowers emerge for the season to add to her Container Garden. She has some idea each year looking intently on each of the Garden Catalogs she has done for Decades. When she makes her yearly order, or, when we go to the various stores to pick out her new seeds for the year, it is like we've done a good deed and cleansed our souls for more neat things to do in Life. We love Flowers. Place something on your Dining Table and Bathroom and the World is right! I drive by the various stores and look at all the bright new colors coming in each year. It marks the time for rebirth, newness in one's soul, and makes for a pretty good day for the new.

Mashing the prescriptions and hear a mix.

Prescriptions come in various sizes, colors, and mixes. Some could interact with each other and you need to go over any new prescriptions with your Doctor and Pharmacist. Doubling the effort is all right. Folks get busy and you can't let any margin of error happen because that could cause many problems or even Death. Be careful.

Some are size of horse pills. Who do the pharmacy companies think they are helping---horses! Where are the 'people' sized doses. One medication that my Mom needed, we got out the small butcher block panel, a small

Hammer, the pill cutter, a cloth for the kitchen table and just hammered away. I got out a pill bottle that has the days of a week listed and ready to put a crushed prescription in the different slots. I pounded away. The pill was too big, it has a coating on it that we didn't know that outside covering actually helps relieve acid in the stomach. And, after the third week, we found out it comes in a mix form if requested. So, Mom now has the mix form and the horse sized pills for me to keep crunching til they are all used. Now, the coating seems to be like a fingernail shell that is hard and makes you wonder how folks would digest it. I just keep pounding til all of it is used up. Again, how many Pharmaceutical companies actually realize that the throats of Folks as they age get smaller. And, if they have a mucous inside the throat area, that doesn't help swallowing. So, there is a lot that Pharmaceutical folks need to be aware of.   Possibly, they need to do Study Groups to find out what the aged folks are going through, whether it is their Product or not.

There are so many issues that are there from aging. In my Opinion, how Folks can take their medications should be an important part of what any Pharmaceutical company should be aware of and interested in how their product can be swallowed or even taken.

Enough of the soap box. Excuse me. I have some crushing of some pills to do at the moment!

Use the MyChart, or MyHealth, whatever is provided.

I like this service. It is one of my Favorite situations to help my Mom and her Medical records and Doctor care. You can sign up easily if your Hospital uses this service. I'd say that most places use some various type of this service. You have an Account, go in there every so often or when prompted for messages and information on your care. My Mom has been able to rectify medications, made any extra appointment needed, received information of her Tests which is a Great service, and she can keep up with her Appointments or change them. It is like having a

Medical Assistant just for my Mom. I use this also. If you don't like Computers, find someone to help. They receive the comments or information, and help to send back any responses or Questions to your Doctor and their staff.

In today's world, you need to streamline, make the information flow simplier, and be able to reach your doctor. Email them on this service and know that sooner or later you will reach some staff member and they can help you as fast as they can. I love this service. It keeps everyone aware of any needs or process of your Health care.

Bravo! To whoever came up with this gem. It is worth its weight in Gold. Learn how to use it, check the actual website every so often and watch for your emails when messages are sent to you.

When you outgrow the Family Physician make changes……………….possibly, a Senior Internalist.

People are getting older and there are more of them. Doctors are getting short in numbers and more medical schools are working to help that.

In the meantime, you have to do what is right for the Health and care of the one you are looking after. My Mom's Doctor of ten years, who she really liked and appreciated, was changing with the times. The way the practice was being done, the invoicing, everything was changing. So, I took my Mom to the ER one time, soon after not being able to get into the Doctor Office as originally done, and was advised to see an Internalist who mostly helps Seniors. That was Magic. It allowed her to be with someone who understood someone her age, was patient with that aged folks, and, allowed her to feel she was getting the care she needed at this phase in Life. I am pleased. She had a Great former Doctor, but, it was time to move forward. The Moral: be willing to change Doctors when time and when needed.

Get past the label aging.

Look, what is Old Age. Is it at the age of 50, the age of 55, 65, or, the age of 70, 85, what is it.

Hey, some folks didn't get this far in Life.

We have a Family friend that is 92 years old. His wife passed away and was the Love of his Life. Well, he didn't stop living. He changed, recharged, had Heart Surgery, has a good Lady Friend that comes from out of the Nation to visit once or twice a year, and, takes younger ladies to Dinner, Concerts, or Events. He has kept on going.

My Mom doesn't look her age. She looks ten years younger. She surrounds herself with younger people, sure, her Best Friend is 90 and has another Friend from out of town, the others have all passed away. So, she keeps active with younger folks and the male Friends still alive. Keep active. Keep alive. Keep doing things that make you feel alive. If you need to dress up! then, do that. Look Great! If you need to throw a small party or Dinner for some Friends, then, do that.

Don't paint yourself or the ones you are caring for into a corner that just fits what the rest of the World is dishing out. Explore no ventures, look toward new adventures, learn to play Chess, learn to do Shuffleboard contests, go to more BINGO, Volunteer for the local Schools to mentor, date someone 20 years younger, or, at least 10 years younger, go do Speed Dating, go on Vacation Tours for Singles, take a Baking Class, go to a local University or College and see FREE Events.   There are so many new things you can do. Sure, some Cliff diving or Parasailing may be out of the picture, but, don't be defined, confined, or, stuck in some corner. Break out of the ordinary and be extraordinary.

My Mom doesn't think how to NOT be active, to NOT expand her horizons, she is UP to what new comes around and what NEW can be done. Sure, on

Computers she isn't shining too brightly....even with a new Kindle she just got from my Brother, but, she is at least reading about it. And, it is going to open up even more of the World to her.   Go after Life, some can not. Be Grateful.

Celebrate Life! At any condition. You aren't Dead, yet! And, who told you that you were!

No matter what a person has going on with their Health, if you are still alive, it is a Good Day! So, why not Celebrate! Every day that you are living.

There is usually someone else going through something worse than what you are going through. Sometimes, not, but, most times they are. So, do what you can to get your Health, or, the one you are caring for, to be better. It may take weeks, months, or a few years.

Life can be Celebrated! With a small cake from the Bakery one Friday, see some Movies on TV from renting from the Library or your favorite store, have a nice Lunch at a favorite restaurant once a month, or, what you can afford, again, Dress Up! and feel good about yourself. Put some Flowers on the Table or in the Bathroom. Life is for the living! So, find ways to keep things going forward. It isn't wrong to smile, laugh, and dance.

Follow the Doctor's instructions, you aren't a M.D.

When the Doctor states a certain type of care to be done, do follow it. Sure, there are times you need to take things in your own hands, and, that happens, but, do follow after Surgery instructions, call the Doctor Office if ever needed, and if you have a "My Chart" or some "Hospital named Chart" that is always a Great resource for you, and, the ER is always a call away. Don't be afraid to go to the ER. They have trauma Doctors that are usually hard to beat. They are thorough and know pretty fast what conditions are and what needs to be done. Impressive is what I've found at a Hospital ER. Again, follow what they say. It is to save a Life, continue a Life, and to become a Solution to a problem. If you have Questions, ask the Doctor. Understand why and what you are having to do. Asking does NOT mean you are stupid, that others will make FUN!!! of you, or, think you are dumb. Who cares. Get the information correctly and definitely what needs to be done. Good Luck! Follow the Doctor orders.

Listen to the Pharmacist and talk to them: interactions of medications.

This is important. Ask the Pharmacist about any interactions with your current Medications. Sure, ask the Doctor, but, go over it with the Pharmacist. People get busy and you want to make sure you can take what you need.

Before more folks were aware of this terrible issue, of Drug interaction, I had a horrible situation with a Realtor. She was helping at an Open House for a House Investment to sell. I stopped by to see how things were going. She all of a sudden felt bad, nauseated, light headed. I thought it was a low blood sugar thing. I asked her to sit down on the kitchen floor, since there was no furniture in the House, and I raced to get some cola and peanut butter crackers from my car. She stated she felt better afterward and seemed stronger and more coherent. We talked for a bit about several things. It was like she was mentoring me in a fast, factual, and caring manner. It was very striking at the moment, like a Heaven sent Angel, to be Quite frankly. Sometimes God puts us in situations or infront of people to help us. I was still concerned for her Health. She also told me that she actually fainted a week or so before and had just changed her High Blood pressure medicine. Well, when we both left I did leave a message with the Owner of the Realtor company what had happened. I left two messages to make sure someone knew what went on. About a couple of weeks later, or less, the Realtor passed away. She was a kind, older Lady, a real Lady of grace, and was in her Industry for a long time. I was saddened that a nice Lady like her had passed away. I was told it was evidently the Drugs she was taking interacted badly with each other. Possibly, she didn't watch for the signs, didn't know to ask the Doctor to change the medication or the dosage amount. Either way, it was sad that she, and many more at that time were passing away. In the USA, it was becoming more common place.

So, with my Mom, we watch dosage, what interacts with other medicines and how. We are very diligent on this knowing what can happen. Don't care what others think. It is your Life, you only live once, and you don't get a second chance, usually. Be the BEST Health Advocate for yourself and the one that you are Caregiving. It matters.

Sometimes it is Life or Death.

Looking Good for Others and Yourself: Dress Up!

I can't overstate this enough. Dress Up! once in a while. Use the clothes you have. So you don't go to many Music Concerts anymore..........use that neat Jacket and go to Lunch with someone. Use those shoes for another type situation. Use your Jewelry going to the Library or when walking around the Mall. Or, wear them when Grocery Shopping. I say, use the items you have. Dust off those Handbags and make an outfit Sizzle. Wear some neat ensembles to the Beauty Shop. Simmer and shine! If a male, then use those ties and look dazzling when going to the Barber or the Bowling

Alley. You just don't know who you may see and who you may meet. Feel Good about yourself, and look marvelous! Feel marvelous.

This may help folks feel better about themselves and want to be somewhere instead of the four walls. Get out and it can be exercising in disguise. But, do use the items in the closet or give them away every so often to someone that will use them.

Curb Appeal.   (watch how high they are…..look for slanted sidewalk spaces)

Some spaces too high up for curbs….my rule of thumb is that if it is near someones knee or as high as their mid calf, in my Opinion it is too high. One of Mom's neighbors actually fell at a local Pharmacy walking down a curb going to his car. He got banged up a bit and some bruising, but, was lucky he didn't hit his head or do more. My Mom is short and some curbs outside of retail or places is too high. I tell her to use the Handicap cut ins and only those to make sure she doesn't fall. He balances out curbs to show she can still function, but, I cringe. One of her Doctors tells her to use my shoulder if needed. She does weigh things out first before getting up on a sidewalk curb. If it could possibly cause a balance issue, she passes on it and goes to the sidewalk cut in area. You can take the extra time to go there also. If you fall, it can change your Life in an instant. Is that really worth it.

You are a Health Advocate for someone else. Also, be your own Health Advocate.

Above all else, do what makes you comfortable. If a Doctor hasn't answered all your Questions or your Question adequately, then, ask again. It is your Body and your Life. Folks get too busy with so much on their plate. Take the time to rest, eat well, and learn to take some time for yourself. If you need a Quick nap, then, take it. Refresh, recharge. You need to make sure that you are doing all right. Otherwise, someone will have to start taking care of you. Always eat enough Fruits and Vegetables. It is nature's way of helping you take care of your

Body. Find out what works for you. I love eating my Yogurt every day. This came from having to have my Mom eat Yogurt from fighting off Bacteria she contracted from a local Hospital. She eats more nuts a day, fresh leafy salad as much as we can. This helps with weight gain, also. We're more conscious of how much needs to be in our system every day. We have always paid attention, but, even more now.

Talk to others about the latest medical trends and methods, look on the internet and piece together the information you think is right and true, and keep informed with the latest medical advances whether by TV, Radio, or the Newspaper.

Communicate with others: Stay Active (you don't have to go home with any of them)

You need to feel relevant in Life. It can be doing only Caregiving. If you want to Volunteer your time with a Non-Profit Group, or, you want to do a part time job, or, you want to spend "x" hours of the day doing your Career, that can happen.

Now, with Caregiving it is very difficult to do a full time Career. It all depends on how much of your time is needed, the severity of the one you are looking after, and what is all involved. If you go to some town meeting or discussion just go there for it being some outlet. You don't have to commit much time, or, go home with anyone. Keep being relevant.

When you can't attend many meetings or events, do attend something. See what others are doing, otherwise, you become outdated and not current. You can look at websites, Facebook discussion and Groups, you can call folks and talk. Don't get bogged down on this. It can be chasing things in the wind. Do become aware of what is out in the World around you. It is too easy to lose touch, have Life whiz by you, and lose what is happening in changes. This can be hard, as your time is gobbled up helping someone else most of the day. Do be open to finding, searching, looking for changes.

Blow the Birthday Candles out!

When possible, Blow the Birthday Candles out and Celebrate another year of ones Life. My Mom gives me the stern 'I don't want to do this childish thing' look and then stares at the lit candle as if it marks something significant. It does. She blows the Candle out and rolls her eyes and says "Thanks". As, we all do. We all made it another year to Celebrate.

Church News, Old News   Keep up with your Church Family, possibly have communion, etc.

One Group of a super resource is a Church Family. It is a Community of the same minded. It is great to have folks to draw from. My Family likes to hear from various social economic lives to see what is going on in the World. Do we all share the same idea of what is going on. You don't have to like another's life or lifestyle. It is hearing if we are all on the same page, does our outlook match or is different from others and what does that mean.

A Church Family can also help you schedule prayer time, it can help have others come and watch over someone you are caring if you have to be somewhere else, it gives a great resource to what is happening at the local Hospital, and possible contacts for Doctors. Mom likes to go to a monthly Medical lecture event to hear out the latest Technology, what causes some medical conditions, and how to treat those conditions.

The Church Family gathered around my Uncle when my Aunt died. They made meals for him to eat during a certain period of time, they made sure someone was calling on him to see if he was all right, they had a wonderful Memorial service at the right time, a month later, that was filled with a lot of Love and gratitude for her Life with them. My Uncle made it through this horrible time much better knowing there were others to reach out when he needed someone to talk. Now, it is how Church folks can get......sure, there were folks already trying to match him up for dating. Yes, already. He resisted and sometimes didn't show up for Church. He didn't need all that, too. He was asked to sing in the Choir to at least have another layer of folks to be around and carve out a new Life without my Aunt. He likes the Choir and taking that one step at a time.

A Church Family is good if it works for you. Don't force it and certainly don't find a Church thinking it will answer all your problems. Hey, some of those Church folks have problems, also. Just have your head on, don't be tempted into things that aren't what you want to do. Take time for yourself to heal. As they say, the first year after a loved ones Death is far better the next year. It is going through the Holidays, the times of the year that were Special, and all those Birthdays. Call your Pastor, Minister, or Rabbi, when you need. Or, you may not. If you have other Friends out of Church they may become the shoulder you need to lean on for a while. Time will heal you. Time will help. Just give it time. Get going forward as you can and when you can. Life does go on. Find the folks you want to travel the next phase

with and keep on going forward. We
only have Today. Learn to live it. A
Day at a time. That is all any of us
have.

Sing in the car Christmas Tunes......even in July!

One time I showed my Mom how the new Radio service that came with her new car, for "x" months til you have to pay for it, works. I showed her many Radio Stations from the BBC, CNN, MSNBC, NBC, CBS, ABC, NPR, well just a sampling. She also got to hear various Radio Stations of a variety of Music: Big Band, Disco, Classical, and lo, and behold, she got to hear some old time Christmas tunes. Her eyes lit up, but, was acting reserve, that these delightful tunes beckoned me to play them. (I was playing them anyway!) I first let her hear some oldies from her era and she liked being in the car singing to some of the tunes she use to Dance with in High School. It was a Fun time. The best she liked were the Christmas tunes. She belted out the songs like a good drunken sailor. The Radio wasn't going to outsing her. She came alive and seemed to enjoy the time singing, like what I use to do with Michael Jackson, Michael McDonald, Patti Austin, Anita Baker, and on, and on. What I really like are the Moments you can play a CD in the car......Christmas tunes in the hot heat of July, roll down the windows and drive along a pretty busy and pedestrian filled street in town. Don't wave, don't let others know you really do realize you are playing Christmas tunes when the heat index is at 110 degrees. Just keep driving along.

Now, Mom enjoyed hearing some of the Christmas tunes that she grew up with, saw on various Variety Shows for the Season. It was Magical. She could feel that in the World there was something she could relate with of her era. So, it does payoff to provide some of the experiences that folks enjoyed in yonder days and years. They remember. It brings them closer to their inner self of who they are, what they are, where they have been, and cherish those fine treasured moments in Life. When you hear the Christmas tunes, grab your Parent or who you are Caregiving and enjoy the music. It can bring back Great memories. Why not remember the times you enjoyed in Life.

Fireworks always look good in the Sky!

My Mom loves to watch Fireworks in the Sky! She loves it when the area neighbors whip out the Big Bags of Fireworks they purchase. She looks like a kid watching all the bright big colors. I love watching her enjoy the Fireworks. It is like watching a kid who is deep into the sight of what lights up the Sky around us. WOW!!! What a thrill.

Why we need those Fruits and Vegetables Like Nature's medicine.

There are many studies that show how much better your body seems to mend itself, nourish itself, and work to help you become better by eating more Fruits and Vegetables. My Family has seen this for many years the Benefits. When My Stepfather was sick, before he passed away, he was already eating a lot of Fruits and Vegetables. The Doctors were amazed how his body fought disease and maintained a good healthy fight. So, we learned many years ago the benefits for eating well.

My Family has always had a Garden and it was just one of the Summer rituals to grow some Fruits and Vegetables. If you rotate what you eat and fix up new recipes or flavorings you can eat a variety, have good nutrition, and allow your body to help fix itself, what it can. There is no Magic wand to fix everything. But, your chances to survive and be well are greatly enhanced eating right.

If you can check your eyes and theirs every year.

Do check your eyes and the one you Caregive once a year, if possible. It will help you be on the front curve of any possible eye disease. It is not that you have to purchase a new set of Glass frames each time, it is just watching that any possible eye diseases don't creep up.

Moisturize.............my Mom even told some ladies before going into a procedure........the Nurses were caught off guard, but, appreciated the advice.

As we get older, it may be time to Moisturize. And, more. Find the product you can use. Ask if you need to help put cream on the backs of arms, or legs, the back, and hands. It is good to keep the Face and neck moisturized. Sure, it helps for dry skin, but, this also helps the person you Caregive feel human. Just a swath of cream on a dry area can wake up the skin, make the person feel that they are very much alive and brings the humane side of things to the table. I help with doing the clipping of toenails, painting them and even using the pumic stone to clear out dry skin on the bottom of the feet. Now, that can make a person come alive and feel that their feet are being well cared for. It may seem small to you, but, to the person having the caregiving it means the world to them to feel a part of the human race. Pamper them. Who knows what interesting things you may discuss, also.

What can you do. Is the Nursing Home the best route for working Children. How do you pay for that!

WOW! This is one of the hardest topics. It all comes down to the Dollars and cents of it. How much time do you have to take care of someone, how much money do you have or insurance, and what is the charge for daily care be it at Home or at a Nursing Home. It is mind boggling what you need to know to help make the best decision. Sure, talk to others, call around, and listen hard to what you are being told.

What to do when you don't know what to do. (talk to someone, anyone that will listen, or, has been in the same boat as you)

Reach out to others. You are not an Island. Sometimes, you may feel you are the only person in the World doing Caregiving, but, you also realize you are not. So, there are plenty of folks to reach out and ask Questions, information, or to find a resource for your particular needs. Don't be an Island. Now, realize everyone has a different experience. So don't judge anyone. Do realize that not all information or answers are going to work for you.

Find out what can work for your situation or circumstance and just keep going from there. Tweak what needs to be redone or added. Don't be afraid to fail, just dust yourself off and restart.

It is easy to feel or look like you are a prisoner. Do remember to do something for yourself once in a while so that you feel that you are still a part of the World. Pamper yourself to a neat meal, or, a manicure. Get a facial, go to the Spa, spend some time learning how to basket weave. I always say, You aren't Dead, yet. Don't get caught up in being "there" for someone all the time. They made it this far without you. So, give yourself some "me" time. It can be "x" minutes or "x" hours a day. But, do make time for yourself. Make that Great Hot Chocolate, or, some wildly wonderful pot of new Coffee or Tea. Indulge once in a while. God put you on the earth to be helpful, to do some mission, and you need to realize you have to take care of "you" every once in a while also.

Don't feel guilty.

Watch your Neighbors, they someday may be YOU!

Our Neighbors are more of an older type since where my Mom lives is for 55 years and older. So, seeing an Ambulance once in a while is although disturbing, it does show that the older folks sometimes need the help. Or, to be taken to the Hospital for further looking into a Medical issue. It is a fact of Life that an Ambulance will be needed. It is like a Russian roulette who will need the service next.

Because more care was needed, several neighbors moved either near to their Adult children, moved in with their children, or moved to a Nursing Home. One couple went there together. The Lady of the house had to sometimes lift her Husband from chair to chair because of him losing his leg strength. Even I was called to come help lift him up to a chair. I'm telling you it was hard for me to do that. He had lost weight, but, it was a heavy dead kind of weight. I couldn't imagine how a 82 year old Lady could have lifted him without some Health issues affecting her also. Well, in time, it did. She also had to go to the Nursing Home. So, when the time came, and the children of the couple got to their senses, the couple was allowed to a new situation, someone else cooking the food, someone else lifting the 88 year old man to and from the bed and chairs, and someone to clean up the room and bed linens. It was tough to see them go, but, it was way overdue. One of their daughters had to take time off her work to make the plans and get ready for the transition.   I'm glad to see it happen. We first called the children when we realized the 82 old Lady was showing signs of being over tired, her memory was challenged, and she just was running out of steam taking care of her sick husband.

If you see that someone needs help, call as fast as you can the children or someone that can help change the situation. We hated to see various neighbors leave but was relieved they were going to be living in better conditions. Also, we were mentally exhausted in what to do in helping these folks but still live our own lives. You can't be everything to others, particularly those who really aren't your Family. The time and strain of caring for others can bring stress to your Life as you caregive for your own Family. Take on only what you can. That is why you must contact other folks Family of what is going on with their lives that you are aware of. Contact them so that no one is hurt, accidents don't happen, and that if anyone needs to be in a Nursing or Assisted Living Home that is where they need to be living.

It is a tough and cut and dried situation, but, it is what it is. Just get to it and be done with it. You can't bring down your Health for others, even if for Family.

Caring doesn't mean that you are consumed by others and what they are needing or wanting. Other folks can sap up your Life if you let them. Don't be suckered by others to help them when they can easily help themselves. Just because someone is older, it doesn't mean they have options of some help from either their own Family, from any paid service, or, of other avenues. Watch out. There are older folks that will test you what you will do to help them. Watch out for the smart manipulative Grandma type. You need to take care of your own

Family.   If it ticks someone off that you aren't helping them or the amount of time you are giving to them, that is Tough.

In Life, there are users and abusers. Don't be near either one, if you can. Folks will give sob stories to cut into your time. Some are legit and some not so much. Learn how to excuse yourself to get back to your Life and the one that you are Caregiving.

Don't be a victim. Help when you can, but, realize that some folks will take from you what they can get by with. Put your guard up every day. Folks can scam the elderly and the elderly can scam you.

The Beauty Shop!

You look Marvelous!

My Mom has been going to the Beauty Shop once a week since a Child. Sure, some weeks she can't make it, but, that is her ritual every week she can make it.

After her time having so many Bacteria she contracted at the Hospital, my Mom wasn't going to miss the Beauty Shop. It gave her a normal schedule, a way to fight the Bacteria. It gave her Hope. Sure, when we went to the Beauty Shop at that time, I brought Alcohol wipes and wiped down each chair she sat in. It was the washing the hair chair, the dryer, the chair she sat in to get her hair done. The first time she came, and Mom looked as pale as any white sheet, under the breath I heard one Lady say "Bless her heart". Yes, it was a Blessing that Mom kept pushing forward. She wanted to have her hair done as it makes most of us feel better when her hair is done. We have Hair curlers for her to use but I sure don't do a good job getting it to curl as well as what she gets at the Beauty Shop. She has been patient with me. I do get better when doing it a second or third time, mostly, in curling her hair and drying her head and not burning her. So, when she visits her Beautician once a week, that is her Therapy and way to keep herself looking sharp, feeling good, and reminding her that Life does go on.

She is Lucky to have a neat Beautician. My Brother and I also go to her. Mom wants to look good and credits her feeling better from her Beautician. THANKS! we all do.

What some good color, some haircuts every so often, and a good perm will do.

Dr. Romelle A. Belmonte, our Saviour

Be aware that you can contract Bacteria even from a Hospital. It is too wild to imagine. A Hospital is suppose to make you well. Sometimes, it can make you sick as a Horse, or, even cause Death.

If you catch Bacteria, Pray that you can catch it before it spreads in your body. My Aunt died from it within two weeks of just having a procedure done. The Bacteria crept down a former broken pelvis bone and just kept on going. She just had one Bacteria issue. Mom was having 5 of them. One did come and go, but, still having even 4 of them in various areas was a challenge.

Our luck in Life, well, God helping us, was this Doctor who zipped up and down the Hospital halls seeing who needed his help. He was very respected in his field. We thought he was delightful. It was a serious moment in my Mom's life. We're talking Life or Death. So, we followed the regime, every day having an infusion, going to either the Hospital or Doctor Office to get that done, meaning a 3 to 6 hour situation every day. I had to schedule others to fill in some days of the week so that I could do the Laundry, work on other things, and possibly, take a nap every so often. You have to be willing to seek the help from others. If you don't how can you take care of someone if you can't even take care of yourself. You won't last long. And, this can affect your health. Learn to take walks, have an activity other than taking care of someone. You are losing part of your Life taking care of someone else. Is it fair? Well, you do what you need to do. But, you need to also look after yourself.

Anyway, after months of going to the Doctor Office to get Transfusions, my Mom finally was able to walk to the Doctor, with her walker, but, made the journey walking on her own as what was the Goal of her and Dr. Belmonte. She made it. Then, she got better and stronger. She finally passed the situation to no longer need an Infusion. That was a Happy Day!

Shortly afterward, Dr. Belmonte died of pancreatic cancer. He made no fuss of having it, you could not see any tears. All we knew was that he was slowly losing weight and we asked if that was intentional. He shrugged it off. We hoped he was doing all right. He wanted the BEST for my Mom and he was a stellar Gentleman and Doctor. We knew he was God sent and hope the BEST for his Family. Sometimes the cards are stacked that there is hardship, some grief, and happiness all rolled into one. Learn to see all the various colors of it and distinguish what you gain from the experience. We are all in this ride on the earth together. Learn to embrace those who want to help you and let them help you. Sometimes you have to ask for help to be strong.

Our Family could not have asked for a better Doctor and feel Blessed. I am so glad that I looked into Dr. Belmonte's eyes and said "Thanks" for helping my Mom. I'm sure he was grateful, but, knew that he could no longer help others like he wanted. I'm sure that was hard on a man full of purpose, full of knowledge, full of knowing he wanted to help more folks. What a Legacy this man has for his Life. Many folks like my Mom who are still here because he worked to save their lives.

Thanks! Dr. Belmonte.

Hobbies can be good.

Do something constructive with your time. Find something for you and the one you are helping to do. It can be knitting, puzzles, Gardening, Shuffleboard, Chess, painting, picture scrap books, and, many more.

One Neighbor knits small afghan blankets for new born babies already meeting family challenges in Life. She maps it out on her kitchen table the design, how many needed, and the colors. During the winter her apartment looks like a retail Market place with stacks of warm small blankets. It is her Mission.

My philosophy is that folks aren't dead til they are dead. Live Life. Make a purpose with your Life. It doesn't have to be monumental. Just enjoy it. Time has value. Enjoy what you are doing, who you are helping, and can you afford it Financially. Don't cut yourself short Financially helping others.

Do find something to give your Life meaning. I find the best way to do that is helping others. Pick up a Hobby you can afford. Is it Golf, Bowling, going to the Horse Races or Casino. What can give your Life some meaning while you can still function. We are all here for a purpose. Find that reason. And, still enjoy some Ping Pong or a nice game of Pool.

It may not be the SuperBowl, but, Golf can be pretty amazing!

If you asked any of our Family who won the SuperBowl, we probably couldn't tell you who even played unless it was the Indianapolis Colts and, or, Peyton Manning. Or, we could tell you who played at intermission. Anything else, we'd not know.

If it was Golf, we may answer your Questions a tad better. Not enough to bet on with anyone, but, would know a lot more information.

Golf teaches you Life lessons. I square up a person pretty much Golf. How they usually conduct themselves in

Golf is pretty much how they conduct themselves in Life. Learn to watch how they treat people, do they cheat, do they make excuses, do they cuss at every whim, do they throw the clubs to the side in a crazy made manner, do they clean up the club head after using it, do they professionally know to rake the sand trap and place the rake politely to the side. What I would see on the Golf course pretty much was how they life life. It was a great indicator to me. My Family has watched Golf on TV for 50 years, I don't get to play much, didn't play much in the past, but, when I did I watched how it was when with anyone else. I learned a lot on the Golf course and hope you learn also when there. Mom watches it from remembering how she use to play. She was good at it. My brother even does some shots better than me. It was relaxing, a challenge to us, and yet, an invigorating way to spend some 'down time' doing a sport we could do.

Mom likes the graceful way the Golfers tee off, and, how they putt and watches how they conduct themselves after making the hole. You can learn a lot from folks in Golf. What sport do you watch on TV or the Computer.

The Kentucky Derby!

It is the first Saturday of the month of May when the Kentucky Derby happens. My Family loves this time of the year. My Grandfather use to own a Department store for 30 years and sold to some of the Horse Trainers who would race in the State of Kentucky at some Race Tracks. Now, the money of Horse Racing back then sure isn't what it is today. But, he did value those loyal customers. When going through Lexington, Kentucky, to my Grandfathers Department store we got to see the changes in the Horse farms. Did they get new fence paint, who added some Horse Exercising equipment, who is adding another

Barn, are there any new Horses that may race in the Kentucky Derby, and, so on. The landscape in Lexington, Kentucky, is the most God-given luxury one can have. The old stone fences there from around the Civil War are stong and stunning. You can feel the history as you zip by in a car. I have the Kentucky Derby on my Calendar marked each year. My Mom sits down and watches the time when the Horses get ready to run the race. I enjoy all the TV coverage of the women's hats, the stylish clothes even the men wear—and, they are getting pretty colorful, lately. Watch out! Ladies! It is all a part of our lives. I remember for at least 50 years how Horses have seamlessly captured our lives for its fancy. There use to be more Ladies scarves, Handbags, Men's ties, watch bands, Hats, and other garmets that you could purchase showing off horse faces or them running in the field. It is such a Fun! spectacle. Louisville, Kentucky, is the BEST possible Host for this event. They exude the typical Southern Charm one expects being below the Mason-Dixon line. For one Saturday a year, we can all live for the moment a cherished time when the World did revolve around Horses, the Celebration of Horses, and seeing all the neat merchandise my Grandfather use to have in his Department store. I'm sure my Mom can hear "how about adding this belt to the outfit. I'll wrap it up for you" as we watch the Horses snap out of the gate and dash to the Finish Line. What a Great Fun! Time!

The Indianapolis 500.

Being in the Midwest and from Indiana, you are well aware of the Great Spectacle in Racing, the Indianapolis 500. Even if you don't like racing you are still aware of this Race. Since we have Family Friends who have either put together Engines and figured out how majestic they are to my Dad who Volunteered for Race Fans to take pictures holding a fake bottled milk and being in a race car. Everyone knows the Greatness of the Indianapolis 500, or, called the INDY 500. I personaly like it when Mari Hulman George, would get up there every year and say the Famous Racing words "Ladies and Gentlemen, Start your Engines!". WOW!!! Now, that was Excitement! Then, you hear the roar of the Engines starting up. Cool. My Mom and I have enjoyed the Indiana State Song for many years sung by Jim Nabors, who played Gomer on The Andy Griffith Show. Now, here in Indiana, Jim Nabors is just as loved and respected as Santa Claus, well, just about. He is one of us. He isn't from Indiana, and lives in Hawaii, but, we count him as one of our own. When he belts out "Back Home Again in Indiana" he is one of us. He no longer will be singing the State Song, and, we are saddened but Happy to have had him around for so long. It will be interesting to see who Mari Hulman George and the rest of the Group choose to sing that. My Mom watches most of the Race, we enjoy it every month of May, also. It is like a Power-Punch month of Great Racing in the Month of May in the Midwest with the INDY 500 and the Kentucky Derby. We're in God's country and that is how it is in this neck of the woods. Great Racing, Great TV coverage, and just a Great time to relax and enjoy Life!

Find something YOU can do or watch that brings things down to a cool calm and allows you to live Life in a slower pace. Let the others Race for a bit. Watch someone else sweat it out. YOU sit and enjoy something to give YOU a time out. It can be the NCAA March Madness, the SuperBowl, the Baseball or Football games, it can be any event you like that takes your mind off things for a while. You need the down time and should find a way to enjoy something. If it a Chess Tournament, some Ping Pong, or a Bowling match, then watch it. Some folks like Boxing to relax them. What makes you happy, do it.

All I can say.

The only thing I can say is that you need to enjoy the ride, some days are pony rides and others are the Rodeo. On Steroids.

It is all right if you need to sit down and cry for a moment. It is all right to call for help and do use that. Schedule others to fill in when you need it. It is all right to Laugh and enjoy! the moments that you can. Not all days are a delightful Parade. And, some days are over the top in what all you have to accomplish. Remember, there is always another day! Tomorrow is on its way and you can finish up things then.

Learn that we only have today, the past is already done and the future belongs to no one. Enjoy! the present and don't assume you will get to enjoy anything an hour from now, a week from now, or a month from now. So, if you want to do it, say it, write it, video tape it, take any pictures, today is the Day! Make the most of each moment, fight through the messy things, and know that if you make a mistake keep going forward. Learn from the mistakes also.

Good Luck! Pray a lot. Do remember to Laugh a lot. God doesn't like sour ones. And, God does have a sense of Humor. Remember that when you start planning out things in your Life.

Good Luck! Keep in there! Cheers!

A Mother Read.

And, Mother Approved Book.

Thanks! Mom!

The End.

Mary K. Hukill lives in the Midwest of the USA.

I like Gardening, watching on TV Golf, Formula One Car Racing, The Indianapolis 500, The Kentucky Derby, watching a Great Movie particularly anything that is good Comedy. Good Music is always GOOD.

Cheers! To Sweet Tea.

CSPAN TV is a Great outlet.

Donate to my Favorite Charity: **American Community Garden Association.**

Have a Great Community Garden Day!

Email: flowersbookseries@gmail.com

www.ingramcontent.com/pod-product-compliance
Lightning Source LLC
Chambersburg PA
CBHW050453290526
45786CB00006B/2272